Table of Contents

Exploring the Phenomenon of Somatic Anxiety: When the Body Talks

Physical Manifestations of Anxiety: Understanding Somatic Symptoms

1. Introduction to Somatic Symptoms of Anxiety

2. The Mind-Body Connection: How Anxiety Manifests Physically

3. Common Physical Symptoms of Anxiety

3.1. Cardiovascular Symptoms

3.2. Respiratory Symptoms

3.3. Gastrointestinal Symptoms

3.4. Neurological Symptoms

Exploring the Phenomenon of Somatic Anxiety: When the Body Talks

1. Introduction to Somatic Anxiety

People talk about the experience of emotional distress in physical terms, and, among its four expressions, somatic anxiety is likely the most common. Somatic anxiety defines the distressing and discomforting anxiety symptoms that humans notice in their bodies. Each of the four expressions of emotional distress contains a component of somatisation, the experience of emotional distress in physical terms. Mental disorders can cause emotional distress, and emotional distress can cause people to behave in unusual ways. The five senses are, by definition, somatic: that is to say, the senses experience things through the body. Anxiety is an unconcerning that prevents no anxiety; for the heavy worry which is trying to impel me to hide behind the proof is none other than the somatic anxiety that separates me more from the circling of the situation. The more I worry about the possibility of additional cancer cells moving from the mosaic into my kidney, the more that itself makes this likelihood more likely. As a consequence, the choice between 'be patient' and 'worry about it all' is actually a choice between 'decay because of the anxiety in my body about my deteriorating health or 'decaying as a consequence of anxiety in my body about my deteriorating health.

This volume aims to provide a comprehensive look at somatic anxiety, when the body talks. The chapters discuss various topics including a broad characterization and the definition of somatic anxiety, historical perspectives of how it has been conceptualized since the conception of history, the mind-body connection, symptoms, assessment and treatment including psychotherapy-based and pharmacological approaches, its impact on daily functioning and physical health, cultural and societal perspectives, and research on some of the underlying mechanisms of somatic anxiety.

Somatic anxiety is to be seen as a specific subtype of the more general concept of anxiety. It is not the same as 'normal' fear or anxiety as experiencing an expected, or culturally accepted, normative reaction to the expected fear-arousing situation. In some actors, extreme hyperactivity rather than "acting skilled" performance can be induced by somatic anxiety. As a consequence, one obvious point is the necessity of early clinical recognition of it for public security reasons. Often this is a matter of proper, timely diagnosis because the possibility of prevention is elusive. An indication of when somatic anxiety days turn into somatic anxiety disorder may be the fact that a person 'normally' spends 25–120 seconds in his "homeostatic" bodily resting position.

In the literature on anxiety, quite some conceptual confusion prevails. Dozens of definitions of anxiety disorder and anxiety exist, which makes it difficult to use one uniform definition in ongoing proceedings in psychiatric, psychological, and forensic clinical practice. To reduce the existing confusion, this study contextualizes and defines somatic anxiety. Somatic anxiety can be characterized as both verbally and nonverbally accessible behavior or, in other words, "When the body talks." Because of intense bodily arousal, medical professionals and psychiatrists working in neurological and oncological settings are forced to do "something" with patients presenting with somatic anxiety.

1.2. Historical Perspectives

Before the so-called "invasion of the mind snatchers" (Freudians) or the movement for pharmakon as therapeia (Neurologists/psychopharmacologists), the only thought or internal mechanism that could manifest in twisted symptoms was the result of some prodigious sin or evil. That is to say, there must have been a foundation laid for internal decay at a spiritual level before the body itself could recall such perversity. In fact, non-occidental psychiatry still holds ancient onto-Gilgamic ethics with slight alterations based on Advaitic principles. Nature proclaimeth and Voila!, genuine moral problems become medical accidents. In the palimpsests of the past, it appears that a certain physician coined the term neurasthenia. Clinicians recognized this state as a disorder characterized by undue physical and mental fatigue and despair, ranging from boredom or dissatisfaction to the incipient destruction of generativity and internal freedom.

Much has been written about the evolution of the term anxiety since its inception. In a relatively short amount of time, the concept has advanced, evolved and aged through various stages of societal conceptions in the Western World. Creeping into our Western lexicon, anxiety at first assumed the odium, sin, and immorality that dignitas had held place over in our Western society for nearly two thousand years. Indeed, the first occurrence of the word anxiety appears to show erasable usage during the beginnings of the Christian Era. Somatic anxiety, as a concept, sprouted up prior to Voltaire's birth in the

Oriental East. The carnal nature of humankind in contrast to the divine counterparts of the inner soul was a point of wonder and exploration for so many philosophers who were arguably the first psychiatrists in the Western world.

2. Understanding the Mind-Body Connection

In this piece, Chen and colleagues have yet opted for an explanation on a most basal level of the phenomenon. Their explanation rests on three levels. Firstly, they describe different psychological models that range from perception-like models to models that describe how bodily signals influence emotions, to misinterpretation of bodily signals in case of illness anxiety and chronic pain. We explicitly encourage them to most vividly describe these processes, as the involved theories lend themselves more to visual exposition than, for instance, beliefs. Secondly, they describe that also on a brain level (that is, in terms of the involved anatomy and physiology) the body and the mind are intricately connected in the process of emotions. So-called autonomic body responses, formerly seen as mere physical expression, have been recognized increasingly to serve an embodied cognition, directing what happens in the brain. In a plethora of research articles surveyed here, basic psychological theories are translated to mechanisms indispensable to steer the neuro laboratory, which were noted extensively before the technical wave of the LBC.

Anxiety is a multidimensional construct that, theoretically and as a result of subjective experience, involves both cognitive and affective components. In contemporary psychology, somatic threats became subject to the spotlight. Somatic anxiety may be the result of different phenomena, from the very basic and evolutionarily given start of a threat reaction in the body, that is, the amygdala, to threat simulation efforts from mid-sized regions in the anterior cingulate cortex to the intricate misinterpretation of bodily sensations on a cognitive level, for instance in panic attacks.

2.1. Psychological Theories

Numerous studies approach the principle of the body's somatic component from various opposing theoretical angles. In broad terms, three main psychological theories may be distinguished, describing how physical body gestures might reveal emotions or anxiety most clearly. James and Lange, or later Zajonc and Russell, implemented the peripheral view of the somatic system, where an individual's physiology is activated first. Whose theory offers us an insight that physical body manifestations (such as blushing) were dependent on our emotions, and there could be no manifestation of emotions without physiology as a foundation are of particular importance in terms of research relating to the physiology of the body in chronic, undifferentiated somatic anxiety disorder that has not yet taken on psychological structures. Ashcraft, as well as Ledoux, are also followers of the peripheral activation theory, holding the view that the unconscious processing of emotion information concerning, for example, anxiety takes place initially and energizes the limbic system (the emotional area of the brain). The physical somatic responses then spread to the individual non-targeted autonomic system and unspecific motor behavior for searching for a source of threat (such as anxiety) in the surroundings.

The importance of investigating the psychological aspects of the mind-body connection in somatic anxiety will go beyond mere medical classification by recognizing somatic anxiety as a distinct phenomenon. Here, the concept of somatic anxiety will be reduced to somatic physical symptoms due to the unavailability of already formed psychological structures. This research dimension will, without doubt, require a closer look at the particular psychological aspect of the phenomenon. The multi-layered approach employed in this latter model can function as a reference point for distinguishing and contemplating various ways of approaching and understanding those particular psychological structures designated as somatic anxiety. The first layer, psychological, focuses on the elaboration and rationalization of somatic anxiety phenomenon in regard to various individual psychological theories. Regardless of the scope (theoretical or practical) it might reach, this research dimension can be seen as an ongoing debate on somatic anxiety.

2.2. Neurobiological Mechanisms

The degree of adaptation involves the use of a plethora of neurotransmitters and hormones acting both in the central nervous system and in the periphery. The main brain functions of somatic anxiety are related to the Aggression System. The cortical-visceral integration necessary for the sense of biological motion derived from the spatio-temporal perception of self-brain movement in the mirror neurons system and from the monitoring of body response planned in the action plan system located in the precuneus-posterior cingulated cortex prompt the insular cortex to body anticipatory response and self vibrotactile alertness. Understanding the parallel organization of motor and premotor circuited preparatory to self and external action represent an important send to the body homunculus located in the superior parietal lobule being the brain spherical coordinates of the body that will be inhabited in the future by the homunculus reflect its imperative of the physiologic action plan. These aspects depending upon right and left superior parietal lobule could be compromised during anxiety disorders including hypochondriac obsession syndrome. In fact, previous neuroimaging studies have shown that the superior parietal lobule, which contained the somatosensory cortex and the somatotopic map of body parts, is altered in anxiety and obsessive-compulsive disorders.

2.2. Neurobiological Mechanisms. The role of physiological changes related to the perception of anxiety disorders is a topic of interest in the last few years. Several findings have shown a bidirectional communication between the mind and the body. In such a bidirectional system, the brain processes are capable of producing changes in the body and vice versa. This fact is essential to understand how somatic anxiety is conceptualized. An alarm reaction is built upon brain stimuli that promote the perception of threat or danger, occurring also due to an unresolved conflict between the cerebral cortex and animal instincts. These are integrated by dedicated structures, including the amygdaloid complex which has plasticity to adapt the degree of alertness to the needs.

3. Symptoms and Manifestations of Somatic Anxiety

Somatic anxiety is likely to link with anticipatory anxiety and in some continuum models, despite being studied predominantly with anxiety disorders, is used as a possible basis for arguments that anxiety and depression may not be as alike as previously thought. More research, however, is needed on which disorders are related with somatic affective disorder processes and are not. The symptoms of anxiety also might differ, that what we call somatic in patients with proposed somatoform disorders has some somatic domain differences than what we see in anxiety disorders. Each of the 6 alternatives reflects a possible symptom of somatic anxiety. There is considerable overlap, which is entirely to be expected, between questions. It may be useful to pick a few questions that seem most relevant and understandable if you are pressed for time. The problem may then be continued at the next session. In the case of verbal questions to the patient, do not frame inquiries from the patient or from yourself (since such comments may provide clues to answers).

Somatic anxiety is anxiety with physical symptoms. These physical symptoms can involve all organ systems and range from mild to severe. Evidence suggests that somatic anxiety was strongly linked to neurological conditions, particularly chronic migraines. Somatic symptoms could also be considered a symptom of a range of mental health issues, predominantly anxiety disorders, where feelings of unease and fear are predominant. In post-traumatic stress disorder (PTSD), they are typically linked to the physiological processes which increase somatic anxiety from initially external environmental factors to later internal ongoing intrusive memories and flashbacks, but they remain part of anxiety subsystem processes in many disorders.

3.1. Common Physical Symptoms

Physical symptoms of anxiety are the result of adrenaline stimulation phenotypically being the 'fight or flight' response (also referred to as our 'acute stress response' system). This physiological response occurs with a perception of threat and is related to physical changes arising from muscular tension which releases lactic acid as a by-product. This can result in muscular pains. Breathing affects our acid-base balance in our body. Hyperventilation, which is present in many anxious people at rest, can also result in a significant change in our bodies' carbon dioxide levels. This, in turn, can result in a drop in blood calcium and children with hyperventilation can experience tingling and even spontaneous (non-traumatic) fractures. In contrast to this, our vagal system is a component of our nervous system and arises mainly from our brain stem. The vagal nerve controls the heart, gains control of the gut/abdominal muscles, as well as controls the musculature around our bronchus.

Somatic anxiety, despite a lack of recognition in official psychiatric diagnostic manuals, is often identified through the research literature as a relevant and meaningful construct. Physical symptoms related to somatic anxiety are among the most common presentations of clinical distress when an individual is anxious. Many people are seen with concerns of rapid heart rate, associated chest pains, tingling in various parts of the body, and sweating. These physical symptoms are often the presenting complaint of individuals who then have their diagnosis of somatic anxiety or an anxiety disorder established later. People often seek help for the physical symptoms of anxiety-related distress if these are severe. They may not identify with any affective or cognitive aspects initially, and nor may the health professionals seeing them.

3.2. Somatic Symptoms in Different Anxiety Disorders

Somatic symptoms are also found in generalized anxiety disorder. Several studies show that patients report somatic symptoms such as muscle tension, being easily fatigued, and trouble concentrating as problematic or significant to their quality of life. In this disorder, however, the somatic profile shows little distinctiveness in regards to the quantity of reported symptoms. However, relative to control groups of other anxiety disorders, the only somatic profile to clearly differentiate generalized anxiety disorder is the chronic state of being anxious and the somnolence that tends to come with it. In obsessive-compulsive disorder and post-traumatic stress disorder, somatic symptoms are also found that are related to control. In the case of obsessive-compulsive disorder, the somatic symptom most associated is a lack of energy, likely reflecting the demanding and exhausting nature of the rituals or obsessions.

In panic disorder, which historically has been linked to somatic sensations from the start (such as feelings of restlessness, palpitations, etc.), somatic symptoms are particularly pronounced. The panic patients' somatic focus serves as a focal discourse in Riskind's et al. CII viewpoint of panic disorder, in which patients are seen not only as focusing on sensations but also as caring about these sensations for their own sake. This results in higher levels of somatic manifestation relative to other conditions. Research has shown hypervigilance to fears in somatic sensations in panic patients, manifesting in other somatic syndromes and likely being an etiological element toward hypochondriac and somatization disorder.

4. Assessment and Diagnosis of Somatic Anxiety

Somatic investigations may include laboratory, instrument-based, and neurophysiological steps, and should be performed according to the patient's age, sex, signs, and symptoms. Since the somatic examination has been derived from the bulimic literature, the step-by-step procedure was tested with high fidelity in a population of bulimic patients or with eating disorders. Even if the thoroughness of the neurophysiological step makes it valuable for assessing the consciousness of the patient towards the disorder, some clinicians may skip it due to a lack of experience or adequate setting. The DSM-5 offers a global, bio-psycho-social, and dimensional diagnostic approach. Among comorbid disorders and propaedeutic findings, professionals must consider body weight changes and general appearance, salivary productions and habits, and bodily eating sensations, respectively.

Individuals experiencing somatic anxiety may seek evaluation for an array of physical symptoms that are biologically based despite having no known cause. A comprehensive assessment that includes a clinical interview, self-reports, and physical examination may help the clinician to disqualify complex or severe mental or organic disorders. Then, the aim of the psychiatrist or general practitioner is to bring the patient from a 'somatic' level of communication to a 'psychological' one. In this passage, a comprehensive anamnesis may be crucial because it can build the frame of the story underlying the nervousness. Furthermore, some neuropsychological tests may be suitable to gauge the awareness and severity of secondary somatoform disorder(s) according to DSM-IV-TR in order to take care of the prognosis. A meticulous somatic investigation of the general health status is needed to prevent overlooking the real, somatic pathology as the cause of the nervousness.

Assessment and diagnosis of somatic anxiety

4.1. Clinical Interviews and Self-Reports

The interviewer or questionnaire should explore whether the individual interprets the occurrence of the unusual symptoms as indicating something very wrong with them. This assessment aligns with both the concept of somatosensory amplification and a catastrophic cognitions prospective that the unusual sensations are not harmful, but allow things to proceed, that the symptoms do not mean that the individual is crazy, about to go crazy, or out of control. The Beck Anxiety scale and the State Scale Version of Depression assess anxiety through somatic anxiety symptoms. The BAI has two somatic symptoms, tightness in chest and heart pounding, and 18 cognitive symptoms that account for 5% of the variance across studies, and the SDS has consumption of five somatic symptoms that make up 46% of the symptom endorsements.

Clinical interviews and self-reports. Although no interview or questionnaire has specifically been designed to evaluate the amount of somatic symptoms occurring in response to anxiety attacks, clinicians may assess the extent to which individuals experience panic and anxiety through various strategies. A thorough clinical interview covers somatic symptoms instead of those focusing on cognitions and emotions. Although individuals who are truly phobic often talk about the somatic symptoms such as trembling, abdominal distress, etc., that they experience, a good portion of self-report questionnaires deal exclusively with fear, suggestibility, and feeling tones. Both the clinical interview and self-reports need to assess the extent to which their somatic symptoms are unusual or personally salient to them. Although many individuals respond to the literary materials on blood shifting all around, the individually tailor method stumbles when somebody personally experiences salient vomiting that is unique to their response to blood.

4.2. Physical Examinations and Diagnostic Tools

Hyperexpression is also seen in patients experiencing an exogenous exposure to an emotion-provoking situation. As a therapeutic aid, the model should display the relaxation over time with repeated exposures to the emotion-provoking situation and the overlapping of facial expression of e.g. sadness and shame suitable to differentiate these two facially expressed emotional states. Normative data for intensity, contextual, and temporal resolution remain to be collected as well.

In the search for an easily accessible so-called biomarker, some approaches concentrate on the serum level or expression pattern from hair follicles for the stress hormone cortisol. A physiological model or high-quality 3D facial expression synthesis as a diagnostic aid should be able to display multiple changes suggestive of autonomic activation, endocrine activation, and brainstem or superior brain processing depending on the emotional state and the time since last anxious experience or in the situation of a chronic anxious disease.

Magnetic resonance imaging in a cross-sectional or prospective study design has not been used in a single study, although it has shown its capability to differentiate emotional states like sadness and neutral states, a stressor from the absence of a stressor.

Psychometric questionnaires with a non-invasive character and stress-induced quantifying salient states can be performed in this context as well. Clinical scores for DSM or ICD compatible diagnosis can be complemented by standardized computer-assisted and supervised discrete analysis for pattern revealing.

For this purpose, cardiovascular measurements like blood pressure, heart rate, heart rate variability with EC or ultrashort ECG, or urine catecholamine measurements or pupilometries can interestingly be performed for incidence calculation and often show altered levels for patients with somatization disorder, for patients with so-called functional syndromes, and for patients with somatic anxiety symptoms such as panic disorder.

Specialized groups of specialists with physical and psychiatric education focus on so-called somatoform disorders, where psychological stress appears to dominate the emergence of physical symptoms, psychosomatic medicine, psychoneuroendocrinology, and psychoneuroimmunology. They use neurological or neurological approaches with the aim to first rule out or diagnose brain or spinal cord or cranial nerve pathology, respectively. Second, the systemic function of the autonomous nerve system and of the endocrine system is regularly checked.

Moreover, different physiological systems bodywide may function on altered levels or show changed interaction patterns both within the systems and also with other bodily functions. These systems are regularly included in assessments of patients with suspected somatic anxiety, such as the gastrointestinal system, the cardiovascular system, the musculoskeletal system, and also the skin.

To begin with, in a minority of cases, the presentation of salience-dominated states can be visually extremely obvious. Eyes and face have long been regarded as windows to the mental (and physical) state and the mirror of the soul, and affective disorders have also been connected to changes in facial expression or ocular and eye movement patterns.

Medical specializations dealing with physical complaints use a wide variety of physical examination methods and diagnostic tools. Although currently only touching the surface, some possible diagnostic aids beyond the use of NIRS or the search for specific production or expression patterns are feasible.

5. Treatment Approaches for Somatic Anxiety

These healthy lifestyle recommendations, if followed, will help patients to deal with problems of treatment resistance that are related to: lower levels of physical health (such as having less capacity for physical exercise), higher levels of arousal (reduction of stimulants, increase of relaxing agents), vulnerability to side effects (overuse of tobacco or alcohol, large doses of medication needed to get over a hangover or to deal with withdrawal symptoms), and addiction to pain/sleep medication. Mind-body approaches harness the body's own resources such as relaxation and even the 'feel good' chemicals such as endorphins that come about with physical activity, and thereby build psychological resources. PMR teaches a person to make their body more relaxed such that they feel less in control of any body signals that come with scary thoughts. We use it regularly in the step-by-step treatment of patients who have somatic anxiety and are afraid of brain imaging or central nervous system disease. CBT is only started once PMR tells us the patient has got a hold of their somatic anxiety using this approach.

Treatment approaches for somatic anxiety. Pharmacological interventions typically used for GAD and panic disorder are commonly used in the treatment of somatic anxiety. However, evidence for somatic symptoms is weaker, and the focus is currently on psychological treatments. The most commonly used are selective serotonin reuptake inhibitors (SSRIs), serotonin-noradrenaline reuptake inhibitors (SNRIs), and tricyclic antidepressants. Discontinuation rates in patients tend to be higher for SSRIs than the TCAs. Benzodiazepines, typically a short-term option because of their potential side effects and the development of tolerance, are used as adjunctive treatments for patients with somatic symptom presentations. Cognitive Behaviour Therapy (CBT) is the most evidence-based form of psychotherapy for somatic symptoms. This standardized treatment focuses on the cognitive part (e.g., the presence of catastrophic thoughts that link physiological symptoms to serious illness) and the behavioral part (e.g., helping patients to engage in daily activities even if their body is sending out danger signals). However, commencing or even suggesting therapy can be difficult if a patient's somatic symptoms are severe, multiple investigations have failed to yield a satisfactory explanation, and if the patient is afraid of any loss of control. So-called mind-body approaches (such as progressive muscle relaxation (PMR) or mindfulness), are therefore also important.

5.1. Pharmacological Interventions

Numerous medications have been utilized in the treatment of anxiety disorders and can be examined as a possible pharmacological approach. The selective serotonin reuptake inhibitors (SSRIs) may lead to irritability and activation that are not beneficial for those with somatic anxiety because of signs of increased central nervous system arousal and increased heart rate and respiration. Alprazolam is a medication that may also be emotionally flattening. Often times, the SSRIs are first-line treatments for those with symptoms of somatic anxiety. The benzodiazepines can address symptoms of somatic anxiety and decrease the physiological activation associated with the parasympathetic nervous system. Benzodiazepines at modest doses facilitate the actions of the neurotransmitter gamma-aminobutyric acid (GABA) and reduce alertness. Moreover, benzodiazepines have muscle relaxant, sedative, anxiolytic, and anticonvulsant effects which may benefit those with somatic anxiety-related muscle tension and problems sleeping. Benzodiazepines may be given on an as-needed basis or on a regular schedule. In light of their side effect profiles, benzodiazepines are generally more advantageous when used on a short-term basis (e.g., not more than several months) and in specific situations (e.g., public speaking, air travel, and dental procedures). The SSRIs are also referred to as first-line treatments for anxiety. The symptoms of somatic anxiety may mimic the depressive condition, hypothyroidism, or general medical illness. In such cases, consultation with a psychiatrist is indicated in order to discuss pharmacological modalities for treatment.

Medications may be useful in addressing the physiology involved in somatic anxiety and reducing the activation within the neuroendocrine system (e.g., tachycardia, respiration, neuroendocrine arousal). In turn, those interventions may assist with reducing the recollection of the traumatic memory and thereby allow the cognitive and psychological therapies to be more directive in their efforts with the client in understanding and modifying the meaning associated with the traumatic event.

5.2. Psychotherapy and Mind-Body Techniques

In 1980, Surawy noticed on an empirical basis, which others also had noted, that in the United Kingdom, for example, about 90% of people heavily burdened with 'breakdown-level' anxiety of the so-called endogenous agoraphobia and panic-attacks version of phobia had been able to free themselves from medication, because of cognitive-behavioral therapies. This made her interested in finding out which alternative 'mind-over-the-body' approaches have been uniquely helpful. Doyle has ably described how she used in her anxious patients the arsenal of techniques that target the mind-body; wider 'psychotherapy' considerations help treat somatic anxiety often using alternatives to, or in conjunction with, neuroleptics, while considering the importance of stomach acid in peptic ulcer disease, for example. Psychotherapeutic techniques like imagery could be used to bring about beneficial changes in functioning that further the talking cure, for example encouraging the self-acceptance which is vital.

Psychotherapy and mind-body techniques - incorporated under the rubric of bio-psycho-social approach - help better manage the psychobiological vulnerabilities posed by anxiety and related mental illnesses. Psychotherapy, in particular, helps alleviate the disablement caused by somatic symptoms by removal of cognitive misinterpretations and their healthy replacement. This reduces 'panic-provoking' thoughts turning the vicious cycle of distress and hyperventilation. Psychotherapy and mind-body techniques are primarily based upon cognitive models of emotion and consequence of altered body-brain interactions. They encompass a wide range of treatments which are integrated in this cognitive frame including Weber's Psychophysics Model to intentional perceptual reorganization of both the somatosensory cortices of the brain to retraining in the meditative and interoceptal attention in Alexander's Technique and Simpkins' neurocognitive approach, respectively.

6. Impact of Somatic Anxiety on Daily Functioning

Clinical descriptions of individuals with somatic anxiety stress the intensity and the plethora of somatic sensations, but remark more so on the absence of subjective, felt anxiety states. People with severe somatic anxiety, in fact, often approach their therapist suffering from intense symptoms and seeking medical tests rather than for a reported feeling of anxiety. Their physical symptoms become synonymous with their feeling of distress. They are thus usually convinced that they suffer from serious and undiagnosed somatic disorders, and in severe cases, somatic hypochondria is usually present. The difficulty of recognizing anxious manifestations is an important initial step of the therapeutic process in a pathology that is often diagnosed and treated as a disorder of the body.

Somatic anxiety constitutes the somatic (sensory and motor) and bodily-emotional anxiety states that result from the activity of the autonomic nervous system. The impact of somatic anxiety on life functioning has not been studied in detail compared to other anxiety disorders. But from our clinical observations in high-anxiety neurotics and from qualitative research, we know how somatic anxiety excessively occupies and uses the body. Somatic anxiety acts as a permanent controller of one's body and forces an individual to always be in a state of watchfulness and hyperattention toward one's body. These individuals feel the body as an enemy they must monitor, protect, and normalize in order to avoid anxious arousal. This is the reason why somatic anxiety greatly impairs interpersonal relationships, supports a general perception of the body as a threat, and engenders a feeling of loneliness. Somatic anxiety can restrict social life, work, and free time; it represents an everyday ordeal and can lead to chronicity and chronic fatigue syndrome.

The work of Bezuidenhout, Temple, and Leber (2016) has made obvious the much broader and more complex relationship between anxiety, somatic experiences, and occupational functioning. Indeed, the authors have pointed out that experiences of anxiety, even at a sub-threshold level, have a meaningful impact on people's somatic experiences, work patterns, relationships, and community participation. Apart from the issues outlined above, experiencing unnerving physiological states such as general tension, stomach discomfort, or sleeping difficulties can impact one's usual work patterns, values, and productivity. A range of practical issues can be identified among people who experience anxiety, even at a sub-threshold level. This could hinder one's usual participation in relevant assessment, as such routines are not always feasible and might not reflect how a person normally deals with work-like tasks.

The impact of centralized and sustained somatic anxiety on occupationally functioning has been identified, and the relationship between somatic anxiety levels and work functioning is well documented. It is evident that there is a substantial impact on productivity, with a significant association between low productivity and somatic symptoms being demonstrated. Little is understood, however, in the management of an employee experiencing somatic anxiety and the considerable challenges associated with this. In relation to occupational functioning, it appears that poor familial functioning is exacerbated in the presence of psychological distress, while somatic anxiety three months after injury is significantly associated with incomplete return to endorsement.

Communication disorders. More generally, people could also underestimate the cognitive burden imposed by complete body assessments. In the atmosphere of interpersonal communication, emotional or physiological effects of somatic anxiety are also salient. In general, they imply that when being anxious in the somatic mode it is more difficult for us to talk without a transparent display of this other aspect of our anxiety. Impairment of communication can also occur in facial expressions, for instance when the focus of the anxious perception is more somatic than in cases of more cognitive anxiety—when we are preoccupied with appearance. At the same time, we know also from the work of Feldman Barret that the central nervous system associates bodily behaviors with emotions. Being anxious might make us act and talk as if we were. Social. This line of research is closely connected to concerns in social psychology that may flourish in the somatic school. For example, body posture is a factor that impacts evaluations of participants overarching in an interaction in experimental conditions. In particular, expansive posture enhances dominance and assessment of leader efficacy. Whether posture displays anxiety on a somatic level enters the paradigm of power research. Power and anxiety display a complex relationship. In general, subordinates are more anxious in experimental settings than individuals who are in a dominant position—however, in real life anxiety can again augment the imbalance as is in the case of prison guards suggested earlier in this paper. If your power is on the line, somatic anxiety could increase. However, the rate of anxiety expressed by these nonleaders was much greater physiological arousal came tantamount. Eventually, the ruditas of emotional contagion theory in Husain et al. 9 a reader conversant of puzzles that are to be solved and niches to be seen with direct application to somatic anxiety and its influence.

Interpersonal relationships. Somatic communication takes place also in the context of interpersonal relationships. Stress-related states activate communicative signals of anxiety in their whole somatic manifestation. It doesn't have to be physical touch in order to affect the quality of the aptitude test scores or measure participants' hands' temperature. However, this line of inquiry focuses more on the representation of the other's distress and indicators that allow to evaluate their states, rather than the manifestation in the subjects themselves.

7. Cultural and Societal Perspectives on Somatic Anxiety

People with somatic anxiety often report feeling misunderstood and that their symptoms are minimized due to the belief that they are not legitimate or "real" illnesses. Some common myths include the belief that people with somatic anxiety are faking their illnesses, lying, or hanging on to their symptoms due to unconscious motivation or some secondary gain. These misunderstandings and pejorative attitudes only add to the already acutely felt alienation and lack of support that most people with somatic anxiety experience. In fact, now popular "awareness" campaigns promoting understanding of mental health problems, including stigma, have often neglected people with somatic anxiety. This reinforces the view that somatic anxiety is both a minor or a self-inflicted problem and, taken to the extreme, some believe that people with the diagnosis of somatic anxiety are malingering. Some people believe that because somatic anxiety does not actively involve suicidality or self-harm, it is not a problem worth addressing.

Somatic anxiety appears to be a universal yet culturally shaped experience. What individuals in a particular culture interpret as symptoms of somatic distress or discomfort may be perceived differently by individuals in other cultures. Behaviors and emotional states that are stigmatized or deemed as undesirable or pathological (e.g., crying, interpersonal timidity) are increasingly likely to be noticed by someone with somatic anxiety and interpreted as reflecting their own internal psychological state. Somatic anxiety has long been an accepted phenomenon in Western cultures. In 350 BCE, such states appeared in Western medical texts but usually referred to the hypochondrium (region under the rib cage); this region was considered to be where the seat of the mind was located and where somatic anxiety was thought to play out.

Radomsky et al. argue that focusing on comorbidities through the separation of severity extensions between panic and/or health anxiety constitutes a step forward in the identification of distinctions underlying the differences between anxiety conditions. They offer no explanation, however, about why HEALTH-ANX convicts should 'idiosyncratically' believe that they were dying of a heart attack while having a fit and being suicidal if it was FA. There is a very wide body of modern international research suggesting delusional somatic complaint subgroups should not consistently experience bodily sensations, and when they do, they more usually are not idiosyncratically or delusionally concerned about them.

When the literature moves to consider differences in clinical manifestations between anxiety disorders, much focuses on the somatic presentation of PD. PD patients consistently exhibit elevated rates of interoceptive awareness, concern with bodily sensations, and attribution of their anxiety to physiological symptoms. They also show high rates of both panic, or PA, and health anxiety or hypochondriasis (HEALTH-ANX) (30-73% rates). Radomsky et al. propose that HEALTH-ANX comorbidities should be classified as a specific somatoform disorder or as a variant of panic disorder. Thus, their position accepts that while findings are particularly prominent in PD, they are present in all members of the anxiety disorders family. Panic patients obviously often believe that their breathing problems signpost an imminent heart attack. They are usually, however, educated patients who are not 'illiterate' from a health promotion/disease prevention viewpoint, and many are training to be healthcare professionals or searching for a place outside of crisis-intervention services. As with the PD patients, they simply may not share the FA DP of fear or anxiety. And while their physicians and those of either do not believe them, there is more primal evidence to the effect that they may indeed be delusional.

As with somatization, the literature on somatic symptoms of anxiety shows the heavy influence of Western psychiatric classification system diagnostic criteria. When calm-focused somatic anxiety constructs are employed, these reflect personal feelings of uncertainty, lack of control, threat, worry about making mistakes, frustration, feelings of fear, stress, and apprehension with worrying. Some build in cardiac autonomic dysregulation or suggest that 'anxious arousal' might be characterized by, for example, blood flow patterns or other 'fight or flight' physiological reactions but offer no explanation for why those might not be present in states where lack of control is not experienced as stressful or threatening. Problems such as these underlie our need to carry out research into the potential physiological evidence of somatic anxiety in an FA context. Grabe et al. have used a range of somatization literature to identify 'five consistent patterns' of somatic complaints across large studies and argue that: [1] replications of these patterns can be considered as representative of all anxiety disorders, and [2] although they did not originate in an anxious condition, they are experienced in an exaggerated or inappropriate manner.

Several decades of international and cross-cultural research have shown that different cultures have different ways of expressing and communicating various mental health problems. Anxiety, direction of causality, cultural explanatory models, and the somatic complaints typically reported by individuals showing state and trait anxiety are highly culture-specific. And although anxiety is a near-universal emotional reaction to danger or threat, psychological research seems rarely to consider somatic symptom experience and perception alongside emotional and cognitive explanations.

Somatic anxiety has been a common human experience throughout human history. Despite having a high prevalence, this phenomenon tends to be stigmatized in modern society. Individuals suffering from somatic anxiety may, therefore, avoid talking about their emotions and somatic symptoms, which may perpetuate mental health stigma and discrimination. In contrast, if mental health practitioners are not knowledgeable about somatic anxiety, persons with somatic anxiety may receive incorrect treatment, leading to elevated symptoms and, ultimately, a longer duration of untreated illness. Public stigma, self-stigma, and perceived stigma should be the main targets of anti-stigma initiatives in people suffering from somatic anxiety. These initiatives should aim to reduce deficits in knowledge about somatic anxiety. Given the internalized nature of perceived stigma, action that weakens associations between somatic anxiety and rejection, as well as increasing hope and treatment efficacy perceptions, are especially important in reducing this type of stigma.

In contrast to recognition and acceptance, these misconceptions create stigmatization. Indeed, at first glance, even fellow sufferers and others in the environment may not recognize somatic symptoms as symptoms of anxiety. The parameters of evaluation may generally be more negative and critical in this modern society. All this greatly increases the feeling of suffering and reduces the possibility of contacting. Because if others do not recognize symptoms as such, they cannot provide necessary support;

in addition, things that the person himself has lived in connection with the somatic symptom and which could be significant triggers may partially be overlooked or played down by others. This whole difficult situation requires, of course, to break the circle of this misconceptions and necessities.

8. Research Trends and Future Directions

As so little has been researched on this specialized topic, Airaksinen et al. have reviewed possible evidence from a broader field of research, such as possible risk and maintenance factors for comorbid anxiety and somatic symptom disorder; possible somatic symptoms in anxiety beyond symptom clusters in classical nosologies; and somatic treatments in anxiety. In clinical practice and in the literature, patients and experts observe that anxiety may occur through the body as well. To date, research has shown that 72% to 89% of anxiety patients also report physical complaints. There is mixed support with respect to somatic comorbidities in anxiety disorders being a risk factor and/or a maintenance factor for negative outcomes and reduced functioning. There is a lack of evidence (mechanisms) in the field investigating somatic symptom-related differences between diagnostic classifications and, finally, there is a complete lack of studies investigating the underlying mechanisms of change in top-down treatments, or whether or not these are treatment targets in (CBT) treatments for anxiety. There seems to be an important association between somatic anxiety and treatment outcome, seeing as bottom-up CBT approaches focusing on bodily states seem to be effective in positively affecting somatic symptoms. It is important for future research to investigate whether targeting somatic states in the body results in reduced anxiety symptoms as well.

Airaksinen et al. now introduce the latest trends in research on somatic anxiety. There is increasing clinical interest in somatic phenotypes, driven in part by expanded diagnostic criteria, including somatic symptom disorder, and the World Health Organization's (WHO) ICD-11 reclassification of a number of subtypes of somatopsychic disorders as distinct primary somatic symptom disorders. Somatic anxiety symptoms are common and have been tied to adverse functional, health-related, and emotional outcomes. The dynamic somatic field is continually advancing, laying a diverse foundation for the field of somatopsychology to digest and explore. There are trends both for identifying the impact of somatic anxiety, but also if somatic anxiety can be targeted with separate treatments. Furthermore, Airaksinen et al. perform the first systematic review of therapeutic modalities specifically targeting somatic aspects in patients with an anxiety disorder. Current findings suggest that bottom-up and somatic-targeted treatments could be effective in reducing somatic anxiety. Potential future directions for empirical research in anxiety and somatic symptoms, therefore, include (1) somatic symptomology as a risk and maintenance factor; (2) developmental mechanisms and longitudinal investigations; (3) novel ways to assess somatic symptoms and treatments.

8.1. Current Research Findings

The term 'somatic anxiety', put forward by van Diest et al. and Pollatos et al., is currently the most used term. Pollatos et al. explored the physical aspects of anxiety and how differences between states of target emotions could be explained from an embodied perspective by measuring interoceptive awareness. Pollatos and Schandry hypothesized that physical pain and depression, for example, may be reflected in particular somatic sensations such as tension or heaviness in bodily locations such as the throat or head. The research on somatic anxiety is still in its infancy, although initial findings do suggest that somatic symptoms of anxiety occur during an early state of anxiety.

Traditionally, emotion is understood as a psychological state of 'feeling'. However, recent research suggests that emotional experience also encompasses bodily or somatic sensations. Misri and Kostaras furthered this understanding by investigating how, in the context of breast-cancer patients with anxiety, the experience of somatic symptoms was differentiated from participants' physical health status. These investigations illustrate the current focus of study, which lies in the experience of a physiological anxiety that occurs. A limited number of empirical studies are available that investigate this latter somatic experience in more detail, that is, so-called 'somatic anxiety'. Different terms, such as 'physiological anxiety', 'somatic anxiety', or 'physical anxiety' are used in this research tradition.

Pilot approaches may provide early evidence of promise and further inform future diagnostic strategies and treatment plans. Pilot alternatives include telehealth, patient-centered care in primary health care settings, and the integrated use of individual therapy and group work. It may be soon enough that individuals will present from the context of their socioeconomic status or experience with structural violence rather than with references to adverse early experiences or circumstances, a long-standing diagnostic question. A body of literature focusing on social determinants of health/somatic anxiety is also burgeoning. For now, promising treatments focus on somatic and neurological profiling, drawing upon principles of neurobiology, somatic and emotional regulation, and trauma care and learning.

As the body of literature detailing both the experience and potential avenues for aiding individuals with a diagnosis of somatic anxiety and underlying mechanisms grows, attention must turn to promising approaches for those struggling. Novel psychotherapeutics and addressing social determinants of health may prove useful alongside the extant and traditional methods. Already, somatic therapy modalities have expanded beyond long-used biofeedback, meditation, cognitive-behavioral therapy, and motivational interviewing. The more cutting-edge dialectical behavior therapy (DBT), eye movement desensitization, Fairy Tale model of Structural Dissociation Treatment (BNTeT), and external and internal assistance in recent physiological resource attention strategies (ePARAS) seek to act on the dissociative impairments and attentional priorities and the nervous system and oral neurobiotic system to regulate somatic profiles. Other psychotherapeutic options include narrative therapy and internal family systems for those who find a deeper, more symbolic conceptualization more accessible.

Physical Manifestations of Anxiety: Understanding Somatic Symptoms

1. Introduction to Somatic Symptoms of Anxiety

Despite the diversity between every case of anxiety, several symptoms are more frequently reported. We call these "somatic symptoms," as they primarily impact the body. All of these can occur at nearly any time, but they are often more pronounced during elevated states of anxiety, particularly panic attacks. In this article, we will take a look at many of these somatic symptoms from being generally uncomfortable all the way to being thrown into a full-blown panic attack. Understanding the body's response to anxiety can be a mixed blessing; while it can clear up a couple of perceived mysteries, it may also fuel more worry. Understanding the nature of somatic symptoms can help us predict and interpret our responses to the development of anxiety symptoms. It can mean learning how to control or embrace those symptoms in a more effective way, coming out on top.

Anxiety is something that each of us feels at some point, to some degree. However, maybe not all of us understand exactly how thoroughly anxiety can impact the body. In addition to the psychological strain and discomfort anxiety fosters, it also manifests in a plethora of physical ways. Everyone is different and thus feels anxiety in different ways; our bodies and minds are interconnected in completely unique ways, which is why anxiety can be so complex to understand, and ultimately, to live with.

2. The Mind-Body Connection: How Anxiety Manifests Physically

This review aimed to elucidate the complex relationship between physical conditions manifesting from mental health, as well as the converse. Mainly, the review of anxiety has the potential to derail the medical testing and follow-up specialists. The section title "Muscles and Joints" describes the possibility that anxiety could exacerbate pre-existing chronic pain states. Anxiety's intrusive nature may also affect the scope and severity of sleep disturbances. Anxiety is not limited to a single system - sleep, musculoskeletal - but instead encroaches into a wide array of bodily functions.

It is already well established in the medical field, as well as in popular media, that excessive amounts of stress or anxiety often result in physical symptoms. Uncontrollable shakiness, excessive fatigue, and shortness of breath in the absence of a physical threat are commonly recognized as typical somatic symptoms of anxiety. Similarly, ruminating on an incoming project deadline or reconsidering a botched job interview has the potential to worsen the chronic pain from an old softball injury. As the bridge between mental and physical health, anxiety may serve as a gateway that connects these seemingly separate encounters. While these are just two examples, they showcase the elaborate balance between somatic illness and mental health that is present in almost everyone. Keeping this interplay in mind may assist in enveloping the fund of knowledge that is needed to explain the "it's all in your head" responses commonly parroted when no clear physical cause for the symptoms can be identified.

3. Common Physical Symptoms of Anxiety

Musculoskeletal symptoms: - Stiffness of joints - Muscle weakness - Tremor

Neurological symptoms: - Dizziness - Fainting - Headache - Tingling or numbness

Gastrointestinal symptoms: - Abdominal pain - Diarrhea - Constipation - Frequent urination

Respiratory symptoms: - Asthma - Shortness of breath - Hyperventilation

Cardiovascular symptoms: - Rapid heartbeat - Slow heartbeat - Lowered blood pressure - Raised blood pressure

Most people manifest physiological responses in situations that are perceived as threatening. Approximately 1 in 3 individuals suffer from a somatic symptom caused by severe stress. Anxiety is a common reaction to stress. Continuous anxiety can develop into an anxiety disorder. People with anxiety disorders suffer from psychiatric symptoms such as excessive concern, panic attacks, or phobias. However, it is known that these problems can also lead to strong physical reactions. The brain consists of two parts: a cognitive brain and a somatic brain. The emotional disorder part of the somatic brain is closely related to the psychological part of anxiety and may also be related to the physical responses of anxiety.

It is common for people to exclusively associate anxiety with psychological symptoms, such as panic attacks or excessive worry. What many people are not aware of is that anxiety often manifests itself physically, resulting in various somatic symptoms. Some sources classify a headache as a typical anxiety symptom, while others classify it as a typical psychological symptom. In any case, these physical symptoms can be a symptom of anxiety. However, there are many other possible causes that should be eliminated. In contrast, anxiety can sometimes occur without psychological symptoms.

Our heart rate and our blood pressure are all dynamically related to our emotional state and subsequent anxiety level. When we perceive danger, our brain activates the sympathetic nervous system, which triggers a sequence of biological events. Essentially, our "fight or flight" response turns on, which evolved to provide us with the means of surviving a physical attack from a predator. Cortisol levels surge; blood flow increases; and the heart rate accelerates in order to push more blood to the muscles and other vital organs. No other organ can respond to emotions like the heart. When a wave of distress or excitement knocks a person off his or her emotional feet, the cardiovascular system gets things back on an even keel. Although the instant effects of this system are to get us out of trouble, over time, a large increase in blood pressure can scar the arteries, making it more difficult for blood to travel through them.

The cardiovascular system can be particularly affected by anxiety. Anxiety can cause an increase in blood flow and the secretion of adrenaline and other hormones, which can lead to several different symptoms. The most common cardiovascular symptom of anxiety is palpitations, which is a perceived rapidness and/or forcefulness of the heartbeat. The individual who experiences palpitations may feel as if their heart rate is increasing, decreasing, or stopping altogether. This sensation can be extremely frightening, as the perceived beating of the heart can trigger health anxiety and a corresponding increase in anxiety. Other cardiovascular symptoms may include chest pain, exhaustion, faintness, hyperventilation, shortness of breath, and syncope.

Breathing-related and cardiovascular physical health problems have been more consistently associated with anxiety states, supporting the intuitive association between cardiac vigilance, breath insufficiency, and anxiety sensations. It emerges as an interesting example or symbol of the bidirectional interplay—the idea that one impacts the other. In cases of asthma and panic disorder, research indicates a complex interplay between symptoms such that initial episodes starting either in the lungs or the mind may produce a spiral of panic sensations and bodily symptoms that exacerbate both levels of dysfunction. Common mechanisms identified include increased fear of suffocation, overattention to physical sensations, and subsequent dysfunction in regulating breathing patterns, as well as overuse of medical resources—largely, medications.

Breathlessness is when a person feels unpleasantly aware of his or her breathing. The feeling tends to be of struggling for air, gasping, panting, or chest tightness. It can occur rapidly, as in the overbreathing of hyperventilation, or it might develop more gradually and have a perceived physical cause outside of anxiety (e.g., tight clothing, exercise). Although breathlessness is usually related to other health problems (e.g., asthma, chronic obstructive airway disease), problems with the actuality of breathing are also commonly reported in conjunction with anxiety, even in the absence of any other diagnosable illness.

Hyperventilation is the classic panic symptom. It is widely known in the general public, even if they are unfamiliar with mental health treatments. Hyperventilation is breathing excessively quickly (i.e., over the normal obligatory breathing rate), resulting in reduced carbon dioxide levels in the blood. Recall that these low carbon dioxide levels can create symptoms of dizziness or lightheadedness on their own. A proportion of the general population—somewhere between 20% and 40%, but potentially more—exhibit hypocapnia (low carbon dioxide) without realizing it because of their overbreathing. This may have some implications for resilience or vulnerability to anxiety and panic.

3.3. Gastrointestinal Symptoms

Functional gastrointestinal symptoms, including abdominal pain, bloating, bowel urgency, and diarrhea, are common complaints in clinical practice. Gastrointestinal symptoms play a major role in the somatic manifestations of anxiety disorders. That is, a large subset of anxious individuals experience gastrointestinal symptoms as well as other physical symptoms, and individuals with anxiety disorders are much more likely to have a functional gastrointestinal diagnosis. Indeed, about 50% of individuals who have an anxiety disorder also have one or more functional gastrointestinal disorder. Conversely, many individuals with functional gastrointestinal disorders have notable symptoms of anxiety or a diagnosable anxiety disorder. Gastrointestinal disorders are a primary explanation for many cases of people presenting for medical treatment in which extensive negative workups have been conducted.

Anxiety is a widespread complaint among adults; indeed, up to 35% of individuals are expected to meet the criteria for an anxiety disorder at some stage in their lives. For years, mental health professionals have recognized that anxiety can have a myriad of manifestations in the body. These somatic symptoms (which include heart palpitations, shortness of breath, sweating, and dizziness) are a fundamental aspect of many physical disorders, making it understandable that individuals who experience these symptoms may end up in a specialist's office having completed myriad tests to investigate the cause of these symptoms. At present, there is growing acceptance of the importance of these somatic symptoms and it is therefore increasingly important to better understand the physical manifestations of anxiety.

While some of these symptoms are just unusual coping mechanisms in the face of stress, neurological symptoms are the most concerning. Seizures can happen in people with anxiety disorders, especially in people who have more than one anxiety disorder. Sometimes, it can be hard to recognize a seizure because it may only cause a loss of attention or it can cause brief muscle twitches that are misunderstood as common anxiety tremors, but real seizures are definitely not smooth muscle activity. Anxiety can also mimic some of the effects of stroke to the untrained eye. It is essential to communicate with someone that could potentially be having a real seizure or suffer from one in the future, since it can become life-threatening beyond the fact that it is considerably painful and intrusive.

An anxiety attack can cause a wide variety of symptoms, particularly when certain signals from the brain in response to high levels of anxiety get crossed. This can include headaches, a tight jaw, tremors, or even sudden tingling in the hands, feet, or face. No underlying conditions are needed to experience this, and usually, this is a very stark presentation that alerts people that they are going through a great deal of stress or anxiety. Dizziness and blurred vision are also commonly experienced. Additionally, panic attacks generally bring about the feeling of being removed from oneself or several bodily sensations (such as inability to feel one's limbs, numbness, tingling, and general body aches) that may be alarming.

3.5. Musculoskeletal Symptoms

The idea of an association between anxiety and somatic manifestations has been complemented by numerous authors. In the early 20th century, Mankin and others considered "anxiety" to be "of the greatest importance" with respect to the etiology of musculoskeletal pain. Muscles are the most common site of anxiety-related symptoms with up to 78 percent of individuals affected by such symptoms. However, others have also reported links between anxiety and neck (58 percent), jaw (50 percent), back (50 percent), chest (30 percent), and stomach (20 percent), and joints including low back (64 percent) and knees (40 percent) are other common sites. Anxiety is also significantly correlated with ratings of muscle tenderness and pain intensity. Functionally, individuals with comorbid anxiety and pain suffer greater physical disability and greater impairment in daily life, especially when experiencing arousal and avoidance symptoms. Along these same lines, greater PTSD symptoms have predicted greater physical disability due to both anxiety and pain; this effect was mediated by avoidance/numbing.

Musculoskeletal symptoms represent one of the most common anxiety-related symptoms. Anxiety activates the muscle tension response which, if sustained, often results in chronic musculoskeletal pain. Descriptions of bodily complaints during stress can be found in ancient literature. Hippocrates documented chest and abdominal pain, and Galen and Polybius connected emotional states with these physical findings. However, the connection between anxiety and somatic manifestations of it was lost for centuries. And even up until the late 19th century, there were few reports of the effects of anxiety on the musculoskeletal system, most of which were scarce accounts seen. Gowers began identifying "irritable spine" back in the late 19th century as a "following several years of anxiety and depression" in a variety of cases in which "long suffered from much anxiety and then had some immediate physical strain or sudden shock." His observations led him to conclude that "these painful states were most apt to follow grief or anxiety, next labor."

4. The Impact of Somatic Symptoms on Mental Health

Somatic symptoms have been shown to represent a weightier symptom profile with more risk of overall worse mental health. People with anxiety disorders characterized by higher levels of somatic symptoms also have higher levels of worry and harmful anxiety-related cognitions. A greater number of somatic symptoms has also been shown to predict (worsen) greater levels of anxiety and proneness to suffer from panic disorder in the future. Indeed, some have suggested that people with anxiety attachment characterized by a high level of somatic symptoms have a more severe psychopathology. However, the psychological literature as a whole is in agreement that mental states and bodily states are closely entwined. In order to illustrate this intermix, psychological theorists have advanced the biopsychosocial assumption, which holds that organic, psychological, and environmental influences intertwine in the etiology and management of illness. Hope suggests quite conclusively that mind and body are each a negation of the other; that where physical and mental states repose, each can turn the other to ashes.

Physical ailments frequently manifest as a result of mental unease. You may suffer from headaches, stomach aches, acne, excessive sweating, fatigue, or dizziness when you're anxious. However, as a result of these physical symptoms, mental oncologists or gynecologists would not be those you were referred to. So, what's the issue? That somatic symptoms—particularly those linked to mental health—are frequently dismissed as insignificant is the beginning and end of the issue. In reality, as discussed, these symptoms can have both a causal and consequent effect on mental health. On the one hand, these physical symptoms can be seen as a barrier to mental well-being by providing a quantifiable and verifiable report of actual distress. Contrarily, however, if somatic symptoms are dismissed, then examining or gathering evidence of mental health can become all the more difficult. As such, the relationship between mental and physical distress in anxiety disorders can be viewed as not just parallel but also bi-directional.

5. Differential Diagnosis: Distinguishing Anxiety-Related Symptoms from Other Medical Conditions

Approximately 2/3 of all mental disorders begin with onset of somatic symptoms. This is particularly problematic for Anxiety Disorders. Objective: To address misdiagnoses, current patient ignorance, and provider lack of knowledge of somatic symptoms induced by anxiety disorders in order to improve effective patient-centered care planning. Studies are cited here directly informing diagnosticians that rare training on anxiety somatic symptoms is common outside of psychosomatic medicine studies.

When patients present with somatic complaints or apparent symptoms of anxiety, it is prudent to exclude diagnosable underlying medical conditions. These diagnoses should be pursued even when the symptoms are "CNS" symptoms, for previously mythical non-physical illnesses may emerge as ME, HIV-Related Dementia, and their extremely significant comorbid CNS symptoms vividly emerge. The relatively small number of somatic complaints that remain once medical conditions are appropriately addressed are somatic complaints which give attention to be "anxiety specific" somatic symptoms. Taking the time needed to accurately identify these anxiety shortlist of physical complaints assists with planning and carrying out effective treatment regimens, for physical symptoms of anxiety need to be addressed in any plan of care.

Differential Diagnosis: Distinguishing Anxiety-Related Symptoms from Other Medical Conditions

6. Coping Strategies and Treatment Options for Managing Somatic Symptoms of Anxiety

While many forms of therapy do not directly treat somatic symptoms, many techniques focused on other anxiety symptoms can be useful in reducing them. Dialectical behavior therapy (DBT) has, through its distress tolerance, interpersonal effectiveness, emotion regulation, and mindfulness techniques, shown to reduce stress and distress experienced by its participants. Some mindfulness-based exercises, such as meditation or deep breathing, can provide momentary relief from stress when feeling overwhelmed. Most experts agree that these techniques could also be used in conjunction with other stress-reducing or self-care activities, such as spending time with loved ones, reading, or taking baths. Other stress reduction or relaxation strategies, such as engaging in yoga or physical activities, have the potential to manage anxiety symptoms, and studies have found that social support, time for self-care, regular exercise, or even gardening can be beneficial. Managing somatic symptoms of anxiety can lead to a reduced experience and clinical significance of concern and also offers the benefit of improving physical health overall.

Though coping may seem like a daunting task, managing or treating the physical manifestations of anxiety can address the problems at their source. Studies have found that some interventions, like psychoeducation seminars, group art activities, and exercise, can reduce psychosomatic symptoms in the short term. If you find that somatic symptoms make it difficult to concentrate on homework, participate in relationships, or simply rest as a result of your stress, it can be important to work on managing these symptoms as well.

Engaging in such activities can help to engage those who are not otherwise attempting to manage their anxiety disorder and so help them in other ways. The ACCUK guidelines suggest that the sense of being grounded and connected with themselves and with others, which can be enhanced by the somatic experience of longer-term process group programs, may also help people to grow stronger and manage their anxiety symptoms. Small group psychoeducation for people with long-term physical illnesses (and often anxiety) can reduce their symptoms by around 30%, which suggests there may be value in small groups of people with anxiety meeting for that purpose. These sessions might best be facilitated by a counselor or therapist but could also be facilitated by a peer trainer (see Part E). It might be most effective (and desired by patients) if the sessions take place after appointments with a referring medic or therapist, but prime time may be early evenings or weekends because those are times when the person will be feeling better, relaxed, and able to go out. The use of somatosensory focusing data has been shown to enhance meaningful diagnostic and process understanding, empowering the client to take control of managing their symptoms.

Physical exercise is an effective treatment option for mood and anxiety disorders, protective against future symptoms of anxiety, an essential component in the conceptualization and treatment of anxiety, and linked with fewer side effects of antidepressant medications. This is discussed in Part D.

The range of physical symptoms experienced and extensive somatization in severe anxiety disorders suggest that treatments that provide an explanation of these symptoms in the context of anxiety and approach them as part of the overall anxiety can be helpful. While there are no widely available interventions which do these specific things currently, Tai Chi and Qigong, for example, seek to explain people's symptoms in the context of an Eastern understanding of wellness and balance in the body.

It is important that psychological therapies for anxiety account for the somatic symptoms people are experiencing, but also work to give greater understanding of the features of the anxiety disorder. Chronic health and mental health problems demonstrate clear overlap in terms of disabling symptoms such as fatigue, concentration difficulties, and sleeping disturbance.

6.2. Lifestyle Modifications

Eating nutritious meals, dressing for comfort, sleeping, and showering might assist in improving one's mood generally. If you can, have a relaxing practice such as yoga. Meditation, progressive muscle relaxation, or deep breathing have the potential to also be beneficial. It's essential to focus on general well-being while decreasing these winter symptoms. In addition to emotional health, it's also vital to prioritize physical wellness. Half of one's body can be found in the water. 4. Gentle and consistent exercise: A high level of brisk physical activity has been demonstrated to be beneficial for mental health and decreasing anxiety. However, in the midst of an exceptionally severe season, you may find it tough to exert unnecessary pressure on yourself. The reality is that all sorts of exercising produce endorphins. It isn't essential to engage in vigorous activity. Simply taking a walk, riding a bicycle, or doing low-impact activities like Pilates or yoga may provide peace of mind.

Lifestyle modifications: If you experience these physical symptoms on a regular basis, there may be a benefit in taking measures to decrease them. It is recommended that you work with a therapist or psychiatrist to fully handle anxiety and other mental health problems. However, there are also lifestyle modifications that can aid in decreasing the impact of these symptoms. Regular consumption of water is essential - it is advisable to start small to decrease caffeine and sugar consumption gradually. When you are ready to have fun, it really helps to reduce the amount of alcohol you drink.

6.3. Mindfulness and Meditation Techniques

Beyond the body scan and interoceptive exposure work in this review, a meta-analysis including over 100 studies found a moderated effect of mindfulness interventions (including MBSR, MBCT, and other mindfulness-based practices) in comparison to control conditions on pain. This outcome indicates that, across studies of this substantial magnitude, there is a significant and reproducible manifestation of mindfulness as a pain coping strategy. We theorize that these interventions provide increased conscious focus on the body, which may reduce anxiety by reducing avoidance of somatic symptoms of arousal and giving people a better scope for moving mindfully through their experiences. Thus, interventions that include a focus on bodily sensations may continue to be promising in reducing anxiety through mitigating against somatic symptoms onset.

In this review, using the same dataset, Burke, Howells et al. found that the body scan did not moderate the association between mindfulness and anxiety, indicating that the effect of the body scan was fully mediated by mindfulness. Furthermore, as previously noted, an adjunct approach targeting the body through an interoceptive exposure had a large effect on reducing anxiety in addition to the effect of mindfulness.

Finally, we must consider the coping strategies available to individuals dealing with somatic symptoms. One particularly promising strategy suggested by our results is mindfulness. The body scan intervention used in two studies in this review aims to increase mindfulness awareness of physical sensations throughout the body. When performed alone, it had a moderate-sized effect on increasing mindfulness, which is consistent with previous literature demonstrating medium effects of body scan practice on mindfulness. Notably, the body scan intervention did not have a significant additional impact on anxiety in addition to mindfulness, leading the authors to suggest that its efficacy on anxiety was largely dependent on the increase in mindfulness.

7. Seeking Professional Help: When and How to Consult a Healthcare Provider

Getting therapy for anxiety is slightly harder in India because public mental health services are virtually non-existent. But getting help faster is always better than getting help later, so if comfortable, get a healthcare provider for sure. In this case, securing a healthcare provider is your first priority. If cost is a question, you will have to tell the healthcare provider right away so they will work around it. Be firm on this.

- The palpitations are extremely severe and prolonged, there is breathlessness, blackouts, or fainting as a result of the panic attacks. - The somatic symptoms interfere with daily functioning. - There is any suicidal ideation. Suicidal ideation is a common secondary problem of anxiety and needs to be treated immediately. Do not ignore these thoughts even if they are not severe or pervasive.

Consult a healthcare provider immediately if:

Even though it is not directly about the somatic manifestation of anxiety, the best way to manage these symptoms is to manage the underlying anxiety. This is the only way to stop somatic symptoms from flaring up repeatedly. Regular somatic symptoms also add an additional stress load on the body, and over time, create a Pandora's box of new psychological and physical conditions. Moreover, there are certain levels of anxiety which require medication and counseling.

8. Conclusion: Holistic Approaches to Addressing Anxiety and Somatic Symptoms

There is no ultimate border between mental and physical well-being in the human animal. The psyche is built on neurotransmitters, brain cells (neurons), and structural proteins that can malfunction on a variety of levels impacting an individual's cognitive, emotional, and physical health. The psyche is also built around personal experience, memories, rational and irrational thought, feeling, and judgment. These are central to mental health and are anchored to the biology of the body in essential ways. Mutual interaction between the body and the mind drives functional changes in stress and change in behavior, the subjective emotional state, and ultimately health. The very new and the very ancient aspects of the psyche and technology are blended in ways that should not and cannot be teased apart. Knowledge of the bodily and emotional person is the path, and the brain and the mind are vital, indeed: the structure of a person's personal contact and embedded biological systems.

At its core, anxiety is not just an issue of the mind; it is an issue of the body as well. The fear and dread associated with this condition can manifest in specific and debilitating somatic symptoms. These symptoms can be nearly as severe as those of medical conditions, and they should be addressed as such. Fortunately, anxiety (and somatic anxiety in particular) is treatable through a combination of medication, therapy, and/or lifestyle approaches. Because the symptoms are so widespread, understanding and treating this important medical condition, particularly psychiatrists and other physicians who provide much of the primary mental health care in the United States, must be formulated on a fundamentally holistic and integrated basis. Mind and body are not merely neighbors; they are interconnected in many ways, and they strongly influence each other. A comprehensive understanding of the distress in dealing with anxiety somatic symptoms must be fully appreciated in order to best address them. Moreover, in order to form an impression that truly in a long-term, fundamental manner, in order to meaningfully blunt the power of stress, it is essential to recognize the totality of the body-mind conflict.